The 10-Day Pure Body Plan

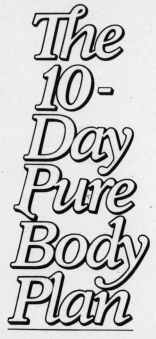

The 10-Day Pure Body Plan

Detoxify Your Body for Natural Health and Vitality

Leslie Kenton

PUBLISHED BY POCKET BOOKS NEW YORK

The material in this book is intended for informational purposes only. None of the suggestions or information is meant in any way to be prescriptive. Any attempt to treat illness should come under the direction of a competent physician who is familiar with nutritional therapy. I am only a reporter, although one who has for many years had a profound interest in how to look good and feel great as the years pass. I write in the hope that some of my research may be of use to others who, like myself, want to live long and would like to "die young late in life."

 POCKET BOOKS, a division of Simon & Schuster, Inc., 1230 Avenue of the Americas, New York, N.Y. 10020

Copyright © 1986 by Fisteba A.G.

Cover photograph copyright © 1987 by Mort Engle Studio

Published by arrangement with Fisteba A.G.

Originally published in Great Britain by Century Hutchinson Ltd.

ISBN: 0-671-63438-0

First Pocket Books trade paperback printing January, 1987

10 9 8 7 6 5 4 3 2 1

POCKET and colophon are registered trademarks of Simon & Schuster, Inc.

Printed in the U.S.A.

For Marjorie Orr

ACKNOWLEDGMENTS

The material in this little book owes its existence to the knowledge and willingness to share that knowledge of so many fine doctors and health practitioners that it would be impossible to list them all. That it was ever published is due to the care, diligence and encouragement of Sarah Wallace— an editor whose skill, patience and devotion to her work continues to fill me with the highest respect and gratitude.

Leslie Kenton, Pembrokeshire, 1985

CONTENTS

1

SPRING-CLEANING YOUR BODY

Have you been working too hard and sleeping too little? Have excess pounds begun to creep on? Are you looking or feeling tired and lackluster? Do you need a way to recover from a post-Christmas binge?

Then you would probably benefit from a spring-cleaning. I don't mean carting out boxes of junk from the attic. I mean detoxifying your body to bring it a new sense of vitality and to regenerate all its systems for maximum good looks and energy. You can spend hundreds of hours and thousands of dollars on lotions, potions and treatments to improve the look of your skin, to firm your flesh and to renew your body. But none of these things is likely to bring you the same benefits as simple natural methods for periodic internal spring-cleaning.

Health and Good Looks from Within

Beautiful skin, a firm and healthy body and a clear mind are strongly dependent on your system's being able efficiently and effectively to get rid of toxic materials and the waste products of your bodily metabolism before they have the chance to do damage to cells and tissues, organs and systems. This principle forms the foundation of the long European tradition of natural medicine: Remove whatever obstructions to rapid and near-complete elimination there may be present in the body. Then, thanks to the natural laws of self-healing by which living organisms appear to be constituted, bodily functions will tend to return to normal. The implications of this natural law for good looks, in terms of restoring troubled or ageing skin to its natural beautiful state, firming flesh, eliminating cellulite, and even improving the health and appearance of your hair and nails, are enormous—so enormous in fact that, in our age of pill popping, fragmented mentality and the tendency to look for a quick fix, many people find it hard to believe. That is, until they try it for themselves.

Clearing the Cobwebs

In fact, the human body is magnificently designed to cleanse itself automatically without any thought ever needing to be given to the process. The trouble is that the kind of food and drink most people in the West put into their bodies, the tendency we have to lead stressful but sedentary lives, and the increasing number of pollutants to which we are exposed through the air we breathe and the water we drink have created a situation in which often far more toxins are taken into the body, and far more metabolic wastes produced by it, than we can effectively get rid of. They are stored in the tissues where they lower vitality, encourage the development of degenerative diseases and early aging, and rob your system of nutrients necessary to keep your skin and hair—indeed, your whole body—looking their best.

Dr. Dwight McKee, Medical Director of the International Health Institute put it rather bluntly when he said that "anybody who has lived the mainstream American life for ten or more years has 70 trillion garbage cans for cells." McKee believes, as do a growing number of doctors who are using natural methods for the treatment of cancer and other degenerative illnesses, that our cells are literally chock-full of metabolic and environmental wastes gathered over a lifetime. To live at a high level of health and vitality and to make the most of our potential for good looks we need to get rid of them.

The 10-Day Wonder Diet is an excellent way to begin. But there are other techniques which can also be helpful— ways of destressing, practices to improve your use of oxygen, means of stimulating lymphatic drainage, and even exercise itself. When they are all used together they spring-clean your whole system, smoothing out and firming up your skin and muscles, sloughing off excess pounds, clearing your mind and brightening your spirits.

That is what this book is all about. Read it, and put the techniques into practice. You are likely to experience a most remarkable transformation in how you look and feel even within the short space of 10 days. Used regularly a couple of times a year, the regimen outlined here is an effective tool for encouraging lasting health and good looks in men and women alike. It can also be an excellent stepping-stone to a whole new high-energy lifestyle—one which will last.

2

THE 10-DAY PURE BODY PLAN DAILY SCHEDULE

The first day of your pure body plan should be a Friday. You probably will not immediately experience a mild "cleansing reaction," as explained on p. 52. However, in the event that you do, the weekend will provide the possibility of a less structured schedule. If your schedule makes beginning on the weekend impossible, begin on the day that is least demanding for you.

There is not a strict daily timetable for the 10-Day Pure Body Plan. All the elements should fit into your days conveniently. Only on Day 1, when you should have a salad at 6:00 P.M., and the two-hour wait required after eating before heat bathing every day, should you stick to the suggested time.

Friday

DAY 1 (Pre-Diet Day)

- Deep breathing, 5 minutes (see pp. 44–46); can be done before rising.
- "Wake-up Drink" (see p. 54, "On rising")
- Skin-brushing, 5 minutes (see p. 39)
- Eliminate all stimulants (coffee, tea).
  Eliminate all depressants (alcohol).
  Eliminate cooked carbohydrates (pasta, cereals).
- If you wish to grow your own sprouts for use during the plan, begin today (see pp. 64–67).
- Walk briskly, 45 minutes, or do some other form of exercise (see pp. 35–38).*
- Relaxation technique (see pp. 48–49) (Practice twice daily if desired.)
- 6:00 P.M.: Large raw salad of vegetables and fruits (see pp. 68–70)
- Body heating in the form of sauna or heat bath (see Chapter 7). At this time, choose *one* of these two forms of body heating, and repeat only on designated days.
- One cup of herb tea before bed
- Deep breathing, 5 minutes

---

*If you are not accustomed to this amount of daily exercise, stop before becoming overtired, especially today, and on Days 2 and 3.

Saturday

DAY 2 (Fruit-Fast Day)

- Deep breathing, 5 minutes
- "Wake-up Drink"
- Skin-brushing, 5 minutes
- Breakfast, Lunch, Dinner and snacks
  Begin fruit fast (see pp. 51–52, 54) for fruit preparation). Choose *one* of the fruits listed for all your meals on day 2. (If you wish to switch to a second fruit on same day, wait at least two hours after eating first fruit, preferably at midday.)
- Relaxation technique, 15–20 minutes* (Practice twice if desired.)
- Brisk walking, or other form of exercise, 45 minutes
- Deep breathing, 5 minutes

---

*If you experience any "cleansing reactions," retire to a quiet dark room and rest awhile. (Deep breathing exercise can also be added at this time.)

Sunday

DAY 3 (Fruit-Fast Day)

- Deep breathing, 5 minutes
- "Wake-up Drink"
- Skin-brushing, 5 minutes
- Breakfast, Lunch, Dinner and snacks
  Repeat fruit fast of Day 2, choosing a different fruit.
- Relaxation technique, 15–20 minutes (Practice twice if desired.)
- Brisk walking, or other form of exercise, 45 minutes
- Deep breathing, 5 minutes

Monday

DAY 4 (Replenishing Day)

- Deep breathing, 5 minutes
- "Wake-up Drink"
- Skin-brushing, 5 minutes
- Breakfast:
  Choose one type of fruit, as on Days 2 and 3 (see also p. 55, "Breakfast")*
- Relaxation technique, 15–20 minutes (Practice twice if desired.)
  (These meals may be interchanged)
  Lunch:
  Large raw salad (or crudités) and sprouts (see p. 55, "Lunch")
  Dinner:
  A dish of steamed or stir-fried vegetables (see p. 56, "Dinner"), with a blended raw topping (pp. 71–73)
- Brisk walking, or other form of exercise, 45 minutes
- Heat bath, two hours or more after eating
- Deep breathing, 5 minutes

---

*The fruit choice on Days 4 through 8 does not include bananas.

Tuesday

DAY 5 (Replenishing Day)

- Deep breathing, 5 minutes
- "Wake-up Drink"
- Skin-brushing, 5 minutes
- Meals: Repeat Day 4
- Relaxation technique, 15–20 minutes (Practice twice if desired.)
- Brisk walking, or other form of exercise, 45 minutes
- Deep breathing, 5 minutes

Wednesday

DAY 6 (Replenishing Day)

- Deep breathing, 5 minutes
- "Wake-up Drink"
- Skin-brushing, 5 minutes
- Meals: Repeat Day 5
- Relaxation technique, 15–20 minutes (Practice twice if desired.)
- Brisk walking, or other form of exercise, 45 minutes
- Sauna, two hours or more after eating
- Deep breathing, 5 minutes

Thursday

DAY 7 (Replenishing Day)

- Deep breathing, 5 minutes
- "Wake-up Drink"
- Skin-brushing, 5 minutes
- Meals: Repeat Day 6
- Relaxation technique, 15–20 minutes (Practice twice if desired.)
- Brisk walking, or other form of exercise, 45 minutes
- Heat bath, two hours or more after eating
- Deep breathing, 5 minutes

Friday

DAY 8 (Replenishing Day)

- Deep breathing, 5 minutes
- "Wake-up Drink"
- Skin-brushing, 5 minutes
- Meals: Repeat Day 7
- Relaxation technique, 15–20 minutes (Practice twice if desired.)
- Brisk walking, or other form of exercise, 45 minutes
- Deep breathing, 5 minutes

Saturday

DAY 9 (Reorientation)

- Deep breathing, 5 minutes
- "Wake-up Drink"
- Skin-brushing, 5 minutes
- Breakfast:
  Birchermuesli (see p. 59), with or without yogurt, or a fruit breakfast as on Days 4 through 8 (These meals may be interchanged)
  Lunch: A sprout and vegetable salad as on Days 4 through 8
  Dinner: Crudités or fresh vegetable juice. 4 oz. chicken roasted without skin, or a country soup of beans/grains/lentils (see pp. 74–76); steamed vegetables, brown rice or millet if desired; a green salad; a piece of fresh fruit for dessert (optional)
- Relaxation technique, 15–20 minutes (Practice twice if desired.)
- Brisk walking, or other form of exercise, 45 minutes
- Deep breathing, 5 minutes

Sunday

DAY 10 (Reorientation)

- Deep breathing, 5 minutes
- "Wake-up Drink"
- Skin-brushing, 5 minutes
- Meals: Repeat Day 9
- Relaxation technique, 15–20 minutes (Practice twice if desired.)
- Brisk walking, or other form of exercise, 45 minutes
- Heat bath, two hours or more after eating
- Deep breathing, 5 minutes

3

THE 10-DAY WONDER DIET

The 10-Day Wonder Diet is a spring-cleaning regimen based on wholesome fresh foods, most of which are eaten in their natural state—raw. This is because raw foods have remarkable properties. At famous biologically oriented European clinics such as the Bircher-Benner in Zurich, high-raw diets are used to heal both chronic and acute illnesses. Research at the University of Vienna has shown that uncooked foods improve cellular functioning and so lead to increased overall energy and stamina. This is why raw foods form the basis of regenerative and rejuvenating diets at the world's most exclusive and expensive spas, from the Golden Door in California to Britain's celebrated Shrubland Hall Health Clinic.

Subtle Magic

For someone who's never experienced it before there can seem something magical about the high-raw 10-Day Wonder Diet. A way of eating in which most of your foods are taken raw increases your vitality, makes you look and feel great, and even helps protect your body from both degenerative illnesses and premature aging. Uncooked foods such as fresh crisp vegetables, luscious fruits and natural unprocessed seeds, grains and nuts have a quality of energy which is light yet strong and extraordinarily health-giving. They seem to impart the same sort of lightness and energy to the person eating them. Such foods are the richest natural sources of vitamins and minerals and enzymes—all of which are important for high-level health, as well as fine-quality protein, easily assimilated natural carbohydrates and essential fatty acids. They are also an excellent source of unadulterated natural fiber.

Spending 10 days on the diet helps dissolve and eliminate toxic materials and stored wastes which have formed in various parts of the body, cleanses the digestive system, restores a good acid/alkaline balance to the body and generally stimulates the proper functions of organs and tissues. In short, it puts you through a kind of transformation which leaves you sparkling with vitality. That is why it is this kind of high-raw regimen which has been used in some of Europe's finest clinics for over a hundred years—to cure illness, to increase vitality, to rejuvenate the body, to improve athletic performance, to beautify, and to encourage natural weight loss. Diets like this one keep world-famous health spas making money hand over fist as they take in worn, tired, stressed people and transform them in a fortnight into more energetic, younger looking, better functioning versions of themselves.

Following such a regimen two or three times a year can be enormously helpful in transforming the way you look and feel, reducing excess weight, revitalizing your energies and getting you back on the track for high-level health and vitality. It is particularly useful when over-exposure to central heating or air conditioning in offices and homes, too much (or too little) sunshine, and overindulgence in food and drink (which begets yet more overindulgence) leave you feeling that you need something to shake you out of inertia. The diet is also used in springtime to get you ready for summer vacation clothes and activities and as a revitalization technique—in short, whenever you have been overworked, overstressed or overeating.

Following the 10-Day Wonder Diet can bring you many of the benefits of a well designed spa program. The alternative to it is spending a week at a health farm. Great if you can afford it. But you can do it yourself a lot more easily (not to mention more cheaply) at home.

Slimming Secrets

The 10-Day Wonder Diet works for slimming too—in several ways. First, it supplies your body with the highest complement of nutritional support it can get anywhere, in the form of vitamins, minerals, easily assimilated proteins and essential fatty acids, so that you don't suffer the fatigue often linked with a calorie-restricted diet. Neither do you end up with those dangerous subclinical vitamin deficiency conditions associated with on-again off-again crash regimens. Second, the natural fresh foods used in the meals and recipes are rich in fiber. This is particularly important for dieters since a high-fiber way of eating not only makes you feel full and satisfied but will also help your body stabilize blood-sugar levels and thereby reduce feelings of hunger. Some kinds of fiber, such as pectin, which is found in good quantities in apples and some other fruits, even help detoxify your body of poisonous wastes such as heavy metals like lead and aluminum.

Designed around large quantities of fresh raw vegetables and fruits, the diet offers a further help to dieters thanks to the high potassium content of these foods and to their ability to render the body more alkaline. The by-products of the average American diet—rich in meat, sugar, coffee and processed foods—are highly acidic. Like stress, they tend to increase the acidity of the blood. Taken over a long period of time, such foods can put considerable strain on your body's natural mechanisms for maintaining its proper acid/alkaline balance.

Dieting itself tends to render your blood more acidic because the by-products of fat burning tend to be acid. This can make dieters feel nervous and irritable. The high potassium content of fresh raw vegetables and some fruits and the ability these foods have to alkalize the body help eliminate those unpleasant feelings of strain and nervousness dieters know so well, leaving you feeling well and calm as the pounds melt away.

An End to Cravings

The 10-Day Wonder Diet is great for dieting in another way, too. It helps wipe out the cravings for foods which sometimes seem impossible to resist and which defeat many dieters. You know the kind of thing: you go to the kitchen and reach for a cookie to go with your coffee and then find yourself eating the whole package. This results in your feeling desperately guilty and sensing that you are hopeless and have "no will power." It also results in your trying to cut back on what you eat during the rest of the day to make up for all those extra calories. For many would-be dieters this eventually leads to nutritional deficiencies and chronic fatigue which only make matters worse.

Such cravings, and the kind of uncontrollable eating which they spur, are often the result of a food intolerance— sometimes called a food allergy. As experts in food allergies will tell you, you tend—for complex biochemical reasons— to crave those foods to which you are intolerant or allergic, so that they become a kind of addiction. You simply can't stop eating them once you take a bite or two. This is a common problem—particularly among those who have experienced on-again off-again dieting. The most frequently occurring intolerances center around milk and milk products and wheat. Many people who find losing weight difficult discover that eliminating milk and wheat products from their diet makes all the difference for success.

Staying Lean and Vital

The 10-Day Wonder Diet is helpful in yet another way. The experience of it leads many people quite naturally to increase the number of fiber-rich fresh raw foods in their menus at other times. And the vast majority of people find that when they continue to eat this way they are able quite easily to keep their vitality up and their weight down without ever having to count calories or restrict the quantities they eat of energy-rich foods such as seeds, grains and oils. To anybody who has conscientiously fought (and frequently lost) the battle of the bulge, this can seem almost a miracle. It is not. It is simply a physiological result of the kind of rebalancing which takes place in the body on a high-raw diet.

In my experience about 80 per cent of dieters fall into this category. The other 20 per cent (to which, incidentally, I belong) are only slightly less fortunate. For us to keep excess weight off naturally—should ever extra pounds start to accumulate—all we must do is cut back on the fattier foods such as the seeds and nuts and cheeses and avoid rich salad dressings and sauces, while eating as much as we like of the rest. Then our weight steadily reduces again.

4

LYMPH MAGIC

There are five main eliminative routes in your body—the skin, the lungs, the kidneys, the bowels and the lymphatic system.

None of them is less generally recognized or more important in spring-cleaning the body than your lymphatic system. Yet the state of its health and functioning is still almost completely ignored by most people. Your lymphatic system is not only a major route for the absorption of nutrients from the digestive system into the tissues—which helps keep skin healthy, youthful and glowing—and an important carrier of immune cells which guards your body from damage and illness and prevents degenerative aging, it is also your body's metabolic waste-disposal system. Carrying unwanted proteins and large particles of waste matter which cannot be removed by any other means away from your cells and tissues, it clears away toxins—the by-products of fatigue and of stress, dead cells, fatty globules, pathogenic bacteria, heavy metals, infectious viruses and other assorted debris which your cells cast off. So essential are the waste-eliminating functions of the lymphatic system that without them you would die within 24 hours.

Help for Lymphatics

Doctors working with natural methods of healing insist that a primary cause of fatigue, disease and cell degeneration with its accompanying premature aging is poor circulation of lymph to and from the cells and tissues of the body. The same tradition of natural medicine uses a number of effective techniques designed to stimulate lymphatic functions as a means of healing even quite serious illnesses—ranging from rheumatism or cardiovascular disease to chronic fatigue. These techniques include exercise, skin-brushing, special breathing techniques, heat treatments and exercise. Combined with the 10-Day Wonder Diet, which is designed to detoxify your body and to improve the purity and quality of the lymph—the clear fluid which flows through the lymphatics (lymph vessels)—they are little short of revolutionary in what they can do for your good looks and your good health. They have been known to clear long-standing skin troubles such as acne, improve the look of puffy or aging skin, heighten vitality, banish muscle and joint pain, and aid in the regeneration of the body as a whole.

Making use of these techniques is simple. But first you need to know a little about how the lymphatic system functions and just how important a role its mysterious mechanisms play in promoting health and beauty.

The Silent Sea

Your body is more than 75 percent water. So important is water to the processes of life itself that, according to Nobel Laureate Albert Szent-Györgyi, "Life is water dancing to the tune of solids." A French biologist rather poetically emphasized Szent-Györgyi's observation by saying: "Man is an amphibian. Even the most beautiful woman's body is no more than an aquarium with 50 liters of lukewarm seawater in which trillions of cells live and fight for survival."

Five liters (1.35 gallons) of this "seawater" are to be found in your blood, five in digestive and other secretions, and almost all the rest is in your lymphatic fluid or lymph—sometimes called "white blood." Thanks to the lymph, a ceaseless interchange goes on between your body's trillions of cells and their surrounding interstitial fluids, so that food and oxygen are exchanged and waste products are eliminated from the cells—all through the medium of water. For cells and tissues to be nourished, for them to remain vital, and for your skin and muscles to remain smooth and healthy and firm, this interchange needs to occur without impediment and the water itself needs to be relatively uncontaminated.

In your body, nutrients and oxygen are transported to the tissues and cells via the bloodstream. Arterial pressure forces the blood through tiny capillaries and out into the cells' interstitial spaces to enable the nutrients and oxygen to be exchanged for the wastes which the cells have produced. Here the water or interstitial fluid, now filled with toxic waste, is gathered by tiny lymphatic tubules and then sent back through the lymph vessels to be detoxified.

These lymphatics are a highly organized and elaborate system of ducts and channels which flow all over your body. In fact, almost all the tissues of the body are equipped with lymph channels which drain excess fluid and the wastes which it contains from the interstitial spaces. This opalescent liquid carries the wastes and toxic products from these minute channels into larger lymphatic vessels, on through the lymph nodes, which are located in the groin and under the arm and the neck. The lymph nodes filter the fluid to remove impurities and dead cells; they are also a place where antibodies, which fight infection or toxins, are made. After purification at the nodes, the fluid is returned to the blood.

In this way, the lymphatic system works ceaselessly to clear toxicity and to reduce excess mucus and waste.

Help from Gravity

The microscopic network of these lymph channels resembles the blood capillaries except that it is finer. And the lymph system in many ways is rather like the blood system except that, while the blood system is powered by the action of the heart muscles, the lymphatic system has no such prime mover. Instead, its nourishing, water-balancing and eliminative functions are almost entirely dependent upon gravity and the natural pressure of muscles which occur when you move your body. These muscle contractions and body movements—together with biochemical factors such as whether or not excessive quantities of protein are present in the fluid—keep the lymph flowing and make it possible for the lymphatics to carry out their important task of bodily cleansing.

For good lymphatic functioning—to keep your body free of the buildup of wastes and toxicity—you need to move your muscles vigorously and often. That is why regular brisk exercise, such as taking long walks in comfortable shoes, is so important not only to firm your muscles and strengthen your heart and lungs but also to encourage the steady and effective elimination of wastes from your cells and tissues.

5

MOVE TOWARD ENERGY

If you lead a highly active life and live on a sparse diet of foods which are unprocessed and not too fatty but high in fiber and freshness, then your lymph system is likely to flow freely and your body will continually clean itself effectively. If, however, you tend to be sedentary and to live on the average Western fare, high in fat, protein and processed foods, your lymph system will tend to function poorly and so permit the buildup of toxic waste products in tissues and around joints. This can result in so many problems for good looks that it would be difficult to list them all, from edema—puffiness of skin and limbs, due to water retention, and stiff muscles and joints—to acne, cellulite, and rapid aging or poor tone of the skin as well as degenerative illnesses and early aging.

Exercise is another important key to preserving youth and creating high-level vitality as well as simply feeling good about yourself: did you know, for example, that regular exercise is the best treatment for depression anybody has yet devised? Throughout evolution our bodies have been built to move. It is only in the twentieth century that we have become sedentary "lounge-lizards." As a result of inactivity many people now live with lowered vitality and make themselves vulnerable to the numerous ailments—from osteoporosis to coronary heart disease—in which lack of physical exercise is a major risk factor. Moreover, exercise can do as much good for your mind as it can your body.

And, just in case you think you have to become a marathon runner or do some kind of muscle-straining aerobics to keep fit, you might be surprised to find how simple real fitness can be.

One Step at a Time

Brisk daily walks, for instance, can not only be a lot of fun, they can be a major factor in disease prevention as they help keep your body clean from the inside out. They can also increase your vitality and improve your mental state.

How far? How fast? That depends on how fit you are already. Start slowly if you are not used to exercise, and then gradually—over several weeks if necessary—work up your pace to four miles an hour; that means you will be walking a mile in about 15 minutes. Once you can do that easily you will be able to walk, say, three miles a day in 45 minutes and you'll be getting a very pleasant but effective aerobic workout which will bring you lots of energy and have you feeling great.

Of course, there are other alternatives as well—you could swim or jog or skip or jump on one of the popular new mini-trampolines which are particularly good for stimulating internal spring-cleaning. But each of these things requires special equipment and special places or times to do, whereas walking can be done almost anywhere by anyone without any special training and without spending extra money.

Make a pact with yourself to walk for 45 minutes every day—rain or shine—while you are following the 10-Day Wonder Diet. If you have young children, take them with you in a stroller or baby carriage. Older children can benefit as much from the exercise as you do. If the weather is bad, then just make sure you are all equipped with rainwear or warm clothing. Or you can get up early before anyone else is awake and go out by yourself (this is my favorite time for exercising). If you go out to work, carry your dress shoes with you and wear a comfortable pair of sneakers: take the bus or the subway to within a couple of miles of your workplace and walk from there. You can change back into the dress shoes once you are at work.

Keep Moving to Stay Young

The latest research into age retardation has reported some remarkable findings. It is not a pill, magic potion or some glamorous and expensive youth treatment which can best reverse the long and rather depressing list of changes that have come to be associated with aging, but simple exercise. How much regular aerobic activity you get determines the level of something called your VO_2max.

"VO_2max" is scientific jargon for "maximum oxygen consumption"—the most critical measurement of your body's heart and lung performance. This measurement is something which in most people steadily declines after the age of 30—at a rate of about 1 percent per year—simply because, unlike our primitive ancestors who remained physically active all through their lives, we lead a largely sedentary existence. As a result we appear to age quite rapidly—we experience a decline in cardiovascular and lung fitness, we lose muscle and bone tissue, our skin wrinkles and thins, and we experience a progressive stiffening of the joints. These age-related changes seem to occur at just the rate at which the VO_2max declines in a person.

But what some exciting new studies show is that a decline in VO_2max is not inevitable, and that when an aging person of 35, 55 or even 75 works out regularly they can restore their VO_2max levels to that of someone much younger. When this happens, energy levels increase, parameters of the state of the cardiovascular system such as heartrate, cholesterol levels and blood-lipid levels return to more youthful measures, skin looks younger, high blood pressure decreases, joints regain flexibility, the loss of minerals from the bones is halted, muscle mass increases, fat is lost and even intelligence levels increase.

High Energy that Lasts

Physiologist J. L. Hodgson at Pennsylvania State University has carried out studies which show that when an inactive 70-year-old starts a program of moderate activity he can expect, in effect, to improve his oxygen-transporting ability (VO_2max) by some 15 years. If he then goes on to achieve an athlete's level of conditioning, says Hodgson, he could potentially regain 40 years of VO_2max and experience many of the physical and physiological effects of rejuvenation in the process.

So exceptional is the ability of regular exercise to reverse aging changes that another researcher, Dr. Walter Bortz, was recently led to write in the *Journal of the American Medical Association* that "It seems extremely unlikely that any future drug or physician-oriented technique will approach such a benefit." Bortz began studying the relationship between age-related changes and inactivity as a result of having his own leg in a cast for six weeks. He noticed that when the cast was removed the "withered, stiff and painful leg" looked like it belonged on a body that was 40 years older. He then began researching the subject and found that, by almost every measurement that could be taken, a lack of exercise produced bodily changes which paralleled those associated with aging. Regular sustained physical activity can go a long way toward preventing them.

Herbert de Vries, age expert at the Andrus Gerontology Center at the University of Southern California, has shown in a study involving more than 200 people that men and women of 60 or 70 can become as fit and energetic as people 30 years younger. "Regular exercise quite literally turned back the clock for our volunteers," says de Vries. And, when questioned about what they considered the greatest benefit of their regular exercise programs, his subjects most often answered: greater energy. The fitter you are the more energy you have. It is the "body so unused to activity that tires at the slightest effort," he says.

Rejuvenating Skin

Regular physical exercise—the kind you get if you do 45
minutes of brisk walking, swimming, aerobic workouts, running, jumping or rowing at least four or five times a week—
suffuses the skin with blood, enhances lymphatic functioning, and increases the ability of your body to carry oxygen
and nutrients to the skin's cells and to remove waste products from them. Exercise physiologist James White, of the
University of California at San Diego, carried out an interest-
ing study to discover just how effective exercise can be at
retarding and reversing the effects of aging on skin. Experi-
menting with older women, he paired a group on a program
of jumping using mini-trampolines with a group of sedentary
women and discovered that the exercisers looked younger
and had better skin and coloring and fewer wrinkles than
nonexercisers. White was surprised to find that exercise also
reduces bags under the eyes. Other age-related changes
which physical activity has now been shown to prevent or to
reverse include raised blood pressure, loss of joint flexibility,
sagging tummy, raised cholesterol levels, and the loss of
minerals from bones (which results—particularly in post-
menopausal women—in frequent breakages).

No wonder daily exercise is a *must* on the 10-Day Plan.
And, while 45 minutes a day of an aerobic activity may not
sound as mysterious and romantic as a visit to one of
Europe's glamorous rejuvenation centers, in the long run it is
likely to do you a lot more good. Not to mention save you a
lot of money.

6

BRUSH YOUR SKIN

One of the best techniques for encouraging lymphatic drainage and spring-cleaning your body is known as skin-brushing. It stimulates the movement of interstitial fluids and breaks down congestion in areas where the lymph-flow has become sluggish and toxins have collected. An extraordinarily gentle yet powerful technique, it can with skill be used to relieve puffiness, to smooth the look of your skin, and to stimulate skin vitality.

It can also be used to great advantage in the elimination of cellulite in women—a condition in which a stasis of lymph-flow has concentrated excess proteins, fats and waste materials in certain areas of the body. This eventually results in puckered skin, alterations to connective tissue and distortions of the natural body shape—what the French call *peau d'orange* or cellulite.

I first learned the technique of skin-brushing from a British medical doctor who specialized in the treatment of chronic illnesses by natural means. It consists of spending five minutes a day, before your bath, brushing your skin all over with a natural fiber brush. You begin at the tips of your shoulders and cover your whole body (except the head) with long smooth strokes over the shoulders, arms and trunk in a downward motion, then upward over the feet, legs and hips.

You need only go over your skin once for it to work. How firmly you press depends entirely on how toned your skin and body are now. Go easy to begin with. Your skin will soon become fitter and then you will be able to work far more vigorously over it.

This kind of skin-brushing, done daily, is one of the simplest but most effective treatments for lumpy thighs and hips that you will find anywhere. It does two things. First, it eliminates toxic wastes through the surface of the skin—not only in the specific cellulite areas but all over the body. Second, it stimulates lymphatic drainage all over.

Test for Yourself

Being your body's largest organ and one of the most important for elimination (almost a third of your body's wastes can be eliminated through the skin), skin that is brushed regularly yields up the most amazing quantity of rubbish which can otherwise remain in your body to interfere with cellular metabolism and produce unsightly lumps and bumps.

You can check for yourself just how dramatic is the skin's elimination of wastes by performing a practical experiment with the help of a towel or washcloth: Every day before your bath, brush your skin all over for three to five minutes. Then take a damp washcloth and rub it all over your freshly brushed body. Hang the washcloth up and repeat the process with the same washcloth the next day. After a few days, the smell of the washcloth will be unpleasant because of the quantity of waste products that have come directly through the skin's surface. Just think of how much better off you are without them.

7

FABULOUS FEVER

Another really effective spring-cleaning treatment for your whole body can be heat treatment. Over two thousand years ago the great physician Parmenides said: "Give me a chance to create fever and I will cure any disease." Nowadays, at exclusive health spas in Austria, Switzerland and Germany, many doctors still use the sauna or special hot baths as a part of treatment for a number of long-term ailments. From the point of view of good looks, heat can do much to enhance circulation in the skin and improve its texture, help eliminate cellulite and generally better your morale.

Many specific skin problems—such as acne, for instance, and dull lifeless complexions—are in large part an indication that the body is not eliminating its wastes properly. These wastes build up too much in specific areas of the skin and result in eruptions or a gray, lifeless look to the skin. It is said that theoretically each of us should be able to eat anything we like and stay well so long as our bodies can completely eliminate the toxins we take in. A sauna or heat bath can help do this. But, according to European doctors who specialize in various heat-treatments, it can also do other things which are of benefit to the body. Controlled overheating of the body increases the rate of metabolic processes and acts as a stimulus to the nervous system and the glands. This is believed to be beneficial for the general appearance of skin and it brings a feeling of mental calm and physical vitality. It can also inhibit the growth of viruses and bacteria. Artificially induced perspiration is one of the best means of deep cleansing the body.

The Finns, who are the world experts on the sauna (there is one sauna for every seven people in Finland), increase the beneficial effect of the heat on the skin during the sauna by switching their backs and limbs with birch leaves to further stimulate circulation. They claim that the sauna makes joints and limbs more supple for graceful movement, while it soothes the muscles and refreshes the mind—even increasing one's capacity for work and enjoyment. However, anyone suffering from a serious respiratory ailment or heart disease should use a sauna only on doctor's orders. Similarly, no heat treatment should be given to anyone who is unwell or already has a fever.

How to Sauna

Here are a few guidelines to help you get the most from this superbly relaxing, deep-cleansing treatment which can be a great help to anyone following the 10-Day Plan:

1. Give yourself plenty of time. It will benefit you most if you take a sauna leisurely so that you have time for several sessions in the heat, with short rests in between and a rest of at least 30 minutes, preferably an hour, after you are through.
2. Never take a sauna until at least two hours after a meal and never take a sauna during a juice-fast (although it can be an excellent idea to take a sauna the day *before* you begin a fast or during the 10-Day Diet).
3. Never take a sauna if you have symptoms of any illness.
4. Wear little or nothing in the sauna—a towel wrapped round you is more than enough. The more you have on, the less effective will be the heat treatment.
5. Take off your jewelry and watch. They will become very hot.
6. Stay in the sauna room for only five to fifteen minutes at a stretch. Then plunge into cold water or take a cold shower and rest before going back in again.

7. Don't water the stones during your first session, and be sparing with the moisture you put on in later ones.
8. Lie down in the sauna room, if you can, or sit quietly. Once you are used to the heat you will be able to move to a higher bench.
9. Leave at least half an hour for relaxing at the end; lie down and let your body readjust to the normal temperature of the room. (This is as important as the sauna itself in ensuring that you get all of the benefits from the treatment.)
10. Don't towel yourself dry afterward. Instead, let the air dry your skin naturally. Then you can have a shower.

The Heat Bath

If you don't have access to a sauna you can get a similar effect—in terms of the elimination of waste through the skin and deep relaxation—by taking a carefully regulated hot bath provided your tub is large enough for you to immerse all of your body except your head in it. The bathroom needs to be warm and comfortable.

The temperature of the bath is crucial. It needs to be kept at about 105–110°F (40–43°C)—just a few degrees above normal body temperature. Hotter than this can be enervating to the body. You can use a simple thermometer to check the temperature every five minutes and keep adding hot water to bring it back when it starts to fall.

You need to lie in such a bath for 15 to 20 minutes with just your head sticking out. Then you should get out, quickly wrap yourself in a big towel or a cotton sheet and lie down, covering yourself with a blanket, for another 20 minutes.

On the 10-Day Plan, it is a good idea to take a sauna twice—preferably on Day 1 and Day 6. The heat bath you can take every three days if you wish. But, if at any time you feel very uncomfortable using either technique, get out immediately and try again another time. Never force yourself to "suffer" if the heat is causing any tension in your body or mind.

8

BREATHE OUT

Even the way you breathe can help clear your system of wastes and set you on the road to new vitality and good looks.

While the act of breathing is supplying your cells with the oxygen they need, it is also removing carbon dioxide and wastes from your body. Carbon dioxide is a by-product of oxidation and energy release in your cells. If it were allowed to build up it would poison the cells and eventually kill them. So tiny blood vessels carry away the waste, which is taken in the blood back through the heart to the lungs, where it is eliminated when you breathe out and exchanged for new oxygen when you breathe in. At least that's how it *should* work.

In most people, however, this vital process of taking in necessary oxygen and eliminating poisonous wastes is neither as efficient nor as complete as it should be. This can be due to many things, such as tissue anoxia—lack of oxygen in the tissues—as a result of a diet too high in fats that tend to starve your cells of oxygen, or insufficiencies of iron, vitamin B_{12}, folic acid or vitamin E which can result in anemia. But by far the most common cause is simply poor breathing. Most of us use only half our breathing potential and we expel only half the wastes. So in effect we are only getting half the support for health and good looks from oxygen that we could be getting. And, because we don't exhale fully, when we take in new air the old air that is still in the lungs is sucked deeper into the sacs. This means the oxygen level in the tiny alveoli which supply the body is far lower than it would be if the air

44

they contained were fresh from the outside. Thus the amount of oxygen available to the blood, brain and nerves as well as to the skin and the rest of the body is reduced.

From the point of view of skin health alone this can matter a lot. Seven percent of the oxygen you take in is used directly by your skin. When skin cells don't get all of the oxygen they need they are unable to carry out cell division rapidly and efficiently and the elimination of wastes is impeded, which contributes to more rapid aging of the tissues.

Less than optimum levels of oxygen in your body can also affect the functioning of your brain and nerve cells. In fact there is considerable evidence that many of the mental changes usually associated with old age, such as senility and vagueness of thought, as well as certain physical illnesses can be the result of limited breathing, blockages in the circulatory system or both. Some researchers also believe that the air we breathe may be at least partly responsible for the subtle energy field which appears to surround and pervade the bodies of humans and animals and which changes according to their state of health or disease. On a simpler level, some physicians and breathing therapists, such as the late Captain William Knowles, have had excellent results when treating chronic chest complaints, fatigue, depression and nervous disorders simply by teaching patients the art of breathing fully. Making changes in the way you breathe, using specific methods of breath-control, can not only help detoxify your body but also increase your vitality, calm your emotions when they are disturbed and clear an overtaxed mind. The 10-Day Plan would not be complete without learning how to breathe fully. It is virtually a necessity for high-level well-being and good looks.

The Art of the Full Breath

1. When you breathe, breathe with your whole chest and your abdomen too. Most of us breathe with only the top part of our body, which means we are not fully lowering the diaphragm and expanding the lungs and so are not

making use of our full capacity. This kind of restricted breathing stifles emotional expression and is often linked with anxiety, depression and worry. To check for abdominal breathing, lie flat on the floor or on a firm bed, and put your hands on your tummy. Does it swell when you breathe in and sink when you breathe out? It should. Lying flat on this firm surface, practice breathing fully and gently for five minutes, morning and evening (perhaps before you get out of bed and just before going to sleep), until you get the *feel* of it.

2. Make sure that with each out-breath you let out all the air you have taken in. By exhaling more of the carbon dioxide, you will get rid of more of the cells' waste products and you will be able to make full use of each new breath of air as it is taken down into your lungs.

3. Be sure to get your daily dose of aerobic exercise— walking, jogging, swimming, jumping, cycling, dancing or whatever you prefer. This demands that you make full use of your lungs every day. Lungs need to be stressed daily for peak performance.

4. Use the following exercise for five minutes twice a day to increase your lung capacity, slenderize your middle, purify your blood, and help you learn the art of fuller breathing. You can also use it whenever you feel tense or need to clear your head.

Resting your hands on your ribcage at the sides, just above the waist, breathe out completely. Now inhale gently through the nose, letting your abdomen swell as much as it will to a slow count of five. Continue to breathe in through the nose to another count of five, this time letting your ribs expand under your hands and finally your chest too (but don't raise your sholders in the process). Hold your breath for a count of five, and now let it out through your mouth as you count slowly to ten, noticing how your ribcage shrinks beneath your hands and pulling in with your abdomen until you have released all the air. Repeat four times.

9

DESTRESS NOW

$\mathcal{P}$rolonged and excessive stress can be damaging to health. In no small part this is because almost all of the biochemical substances associated with the stressed state tend to render the system more acid and to cause internal pollution. But stress is by no means all bad. You need stress to live. Without physical and mental challenges you would never feel the excitement, enthusiasm and creative energy which are such an important part of high-level health and vitality. In fact it is not the stress itself which is bad for you. Stress is harmful only if you don't know how to manage it well. That's why an important part of the 10-Day Plan is learning a technique to do just that.

Making a Friend of Stress

Stress and relaxation are really like two sides of the same coin. To make stress work *for* rather than *against* you and to maintain your vitality and health even when things get tough, you need to be able to move at will from the active, dynamic, stressed state into the quiet, restorative, relaxed one and back again. Then stress will become your friend rather than your enemy.

There are lots of ways of doing this. Your exercise program will help, as will your diet, if it is high in natural unprocessed foods. Hobbies can help too, and pleasant walks or listening to music. But perhaps the best way of all of balancing the stress you are exposed to is by learning to turn on your "relaxation response" at will. This you can do by practicing a simple mental exercise for 10 or 15 minutes every morning and evening. In fact you can do this almost anywhere, even on a bus or train on the way to work if you like. Practicing it on the way to and from work gives you a pleasant and effective "stress break." It will have you arriving in a relaxed but energized state, ready for whatever lies ahead of you. This technique was designed by Dr. Herbert Benson, a cardiologist from the Harvard University School of Medicine. Its beneficial results have been thoroughly laboratory-tested. Practiced twice a day, it can relieve inner tensions, lower blood pressure and generally let you turn off the harmful bodily effects of stress. Here's how:

The Relaxation Response

Sitting quietly in a chair where you are not likely to be disturbed, close your eyes.

"Settle in" by letting go of tension in your muscles, starting from your feet and working up to your face.

Now, as you breathe in normally through your nose, be aware of the air entering your body. Don't *force* anything, just *watch* what is happening. As you breathe out say the word "one" silently to yourself. So it goes something like this: in-breath . . . out-breath . . . "one" . . . in-breath . . . out-breath . . . "one." The word doesn't have to be "one"— you can pick any word that appeals to you.

Continue like this for 10 or 15 minutes. Open your eyes briefly to check the time if you want, but don't use an alarm. When you are finished, slowly open your eyes. Then sit still for a minute or so before going back to work or on with whatever you were doing.

Don't worry about how well you are "doing it." Try to keep a passive attitude and let relaxation come at its own pace. If your thoughts distract you, don't worry about them. Just gently bring yourself back to repeating the word silently again.

Practicing such a technique once or twice a day will make the response come gradually more and more easily. It will also help prevent the build-up of the toxic waste products of long-term stress. (But don't do it just after a meal. Your digestive processes can inhibit the relaxation effect.) Ten days of practice while you are on the diet will set you well on your way toward a future in which stress becomes your friend, not your foe. This little technique is something to be used for life.

10

LET'S GET STARTED

$\mathbb{A}$ diet always begins tomorrow. And tomorrow it begins the day after . . . It is so hard to find a diet that will fit into your daily routine that you can put it off forever. The 10-Day Wonder Diet is different. It is designed to begin on a Friday with a pre-diet day and to spread over two weekends and the intervening week. It is also made as convenient as possible so that even if you have a nine-to-five job, or you have to eat at least one of your meals in a restaurant, you can follow it with relative ease.

And remember that the 10-Day Wonder Diet doesn't affect just your body but your mind and spirit too. It is important for the *entire* you.

How and Why It Works

The diet is divided into four parts:

1. a pre-diet day to prepare your body for the elimination process;
2. days 2 and 3, which are fruit-fast days and spur rapid elimination;
3. days 4 to 8, which are replenishing fruit and vegetable days;
4. days 9 and 10—reorientation days to lead you to practice a better way of eating permanently.

Pre-diet Day—Day 1 (Friday)

To prepare your body for the change involved in eating a raw diet, begin on Day 1 by eliminating all stimulants, such as coffee and tea, and all depressants, such as alcohol. Also avoid bread and cooked carbohydrates such as pasta and cereals, and make your last meal of the day a large raw salad of vegetables and fruits. This is a good time to start preparing your home-grown sprouts if you are going to use them; you may be able to buy them in a health food store or supermarket if you prefer.

Preparing Your Sprouts
Sprouts form an important part of the 10-Day Wonder Diet. As they take a few days to germinate, you will need to begin preparing them on Day 1 of the diet, or even before. If they become ready too quickly you can always refrigerate them. (See page 65 for how to grow them.)

Day 1: What to Do
Follow the guidelines outlined above. Have your raw salad early in the evening, say about 6:00 P.M., and then don't have anything else except a cup of herb tea before you go to bed. This gives your system a good 12 hours to start eliminating.

The Fruit-fast—Days 2 and 3 (Saturday and Sunday)

The fruit-fast is one of the best ways of clearing your system quickly. Because the effect is so dramatic you may find that you experience some mild elimination reactions such as a headache, irritability or tiredness at some point within the first three days. For this reason Days 2 and 3 are done at the weekend so that you can rest as you feel necessary.

The fruit-fast is effective in several ways. In a purely physical sense, fruit is mildly laxative and a wonderful intestinal "broom" to sweep your alimentary canal clean.

Also, fruit is alkaline-forming; most stored wastes which are responsible for aches and disease in general are acidic. When your body is given the chance to throw off these wastes, as it is on the 10-Day Plan, they first enter the bloodstream. The alkalinity of the fruit helps to neutralize them so that they are not harmful and can be quickly expelled. In this way you minimize the possibility of any cleansing reactions.

Fruit also has a high potassium content. This is helpful in ridding the system of excess water and edema in the tissues, increasing oxygenation in the cells and raising cell vitality.

Cleansing reactions

Because the effect of eating all-raw foods is so dramatic, it is possible that you may experience one or more cleansing reactions (although many people don't). If you do, there is no need to worry. It is all part of the elimination process. But it is important to acknowledge them. Such reactions can include headaches, muscle or joint pains, sensitivity, tiredness and unsettled emotions. They are due to the rapid mobilization and release of stored toxins and wastes. Should they occur it is best to retire to a quiet, dark room and rest for a while. Also try to get plenty of fresh air—breathing deeply is another way of ridding your body of wastes. During the first two days especially, beware of overtaxing your body by strenuous exercise: it is working very hard to clean and renew itself and therefore just now it doesn't need added strain.

For Days 2 and 3 it is up to you to choose the *single* fruit which you intend to eat throughout the day. Each fruit has its own specific health benefiting properties. I have found that apples, grapes, pineapple, papaya, mango and watermelon are particularly successful. The following notes may help you make your choice:

Apples: Excellent for detoxification—the pectin in apples helps remove impurities from the system. Pectin also helps prevent protein matter in the intestines from putrefying. The high fiber content of apples also makes them great "brooms." Apples are good for strengthening the liver and digestive system and for stimulating body secretions. They are rich in vitamins and minerals.

Grapes: Very effective cleansers for the skin, liver, intestines and kidneys due to their potent properties which counter excessive mucus. Grapes provide a quick source of energy which is easily assimilated and, rich in minerals, they make good blood and cell builders.

Pineapple: Has a high concentration of bromelin, an enzyme which supports the action of hydrochloric acid in your stomach and helps to break down protein wastes in the system. Eating pineapple is also believed to soothe internal inflammation, accelerate tissue repair, regulate the glandular system and clear mucus.

Papaya and mango: These tropical fruits (mango to a lesser degree) contain an enzyme called papain which resembles the enzyme pepsin in the stomach and, like bromelin, helps to break down protein waste in the tissues. Papaya and mango are good for cleansing the alimentary canal and helping digestive disorders. Mangoes are also believed to relieve depression.

Watermelon: A wonderful diuretic and great for washing your system clean. It is used to ease stomach ulcers and high blood pressure and to soothe the intestinal tract. Juice the rind of the watermelon with the seeds and a little flesh and drink it about half an hour before a melon meal to get all the benefit of the chlorophyll-rich skin and vitamin-packed seeds.

One fruit only is eaten throughout the day because this is least taxing for the digestive system. (It is also, incidentally, the best way to lose weight.) If, however, the amount of a certain fruit available is limited you can change fruit mid-day as long as you leave a gap of at least two hours before starting the new fruit. How much fruit you choose to eat is up to you. Eating fruit by itself will *not* make you gain weight. You will find that you need to eat more frequently than usual as fruit is digested very quickly and does not remain in the stomach for more than an hour. You might want to take about four to five fruit meals spread throughout the day (eating continually is tiring for the digestive system), but should you feel hungry at any point, have a fruit snack.

Days 2 and 3: What to Do

On rising: An orange and half a lemon juiced added to spring water in a tall glass, *or* a cup of herb tea with a squeeze of lemon. Lemon verbena or peppermint are very good "wake-up" teas.

First thing in the morning: Skin-brushing (see page 39).

Eat several fruit meals throughout the day. Choose one of the following for Day 1 and a different one for Day 2: apple, grape, pineapple, papaya, mango, watermelon.

You don't have to eat the fruit "straight"—try grating, slicing or dicing and pouring a little of the juice over the fruit in a bowl. Or make a frappé by putting the chilled or partly frozen fruit in a blender, perhaps adding a little water to make it more liquid, plus some crushed ice, and spicing it lightly with cinnamon, allspice, nutmeg or ginger. You can also juice the fruits, although you lose the valuable "bulk" this way, so it is best to drink the juice only once or twice a day and have the whole fruit the rest of the time.

Replenishing—Days 4 to 8 (Monday to Friday)

This part of the diet is designed to allow the elimination process to continue while nourishing your newly cleansed cells with all the nutrients needed to fortify and rebalance your system. The vitamins, minerals and enzymes in the raw vegetables and sprouts will boost sluggish cells into action and vitalize your whole being. It begins with a fruit breakfast (as the entire diet does); this is very important for it encourages the liver (most active early in the day) to continue the rapid elimination of stored wastes. Lunch is basically a large raw salad (or crudités) and sprouts with some seeds or blanched almonds. Dinner is a dish of steamed or stir-fried vegetables with a blended raw topping. (Lunch and dinner are interchangeable depending upon which is more convenient if, say, you eat lunch at work; and even if you have to eat at a restaurant there should be no problem.)

Days 4 to 8: What to Do

Have your wake-up drink and skin-brushing as for Days 2 and 3.

Breakfast: Fruit. Either one fruit or a combination (not bananas). You can make a simple fruit salad dressed with fruit juice, a little honey and spices, or a delicious fruit shake made in the blender—such as a Mango Smoothie, made by combining the flesh of a mango with some freshly squeezed orange juice.

Lunch: A large salad made from raw vegetables. Invent new combinations each day from what you can find at your greengrocer. For instance: grated carrots, beetroot, white/red cabbage, tomatoes, red peppers, sliced mushrooms, celery, watercress, chicory, romaine lettuce, radicchio . . . The possibilities are endless. Top the salad with generous helpings of sprouted seeds, pulses and grains and dress with an olive oil and lemon or cider-vinegar dressing or an avocado or mayonnaise dressing. Complete it with lots of fresh herbs such as basil and parsley. An avocado is an excellent addition to such a salad, which can also be sprinkled with sunflower, pumpkin and sesame seeds—either whole or ground—or a few blanched almonds.

Dinner: Steamed or wok-fried vegetables prepared in a tiny amount of olive oil and cooked for just a few minutes, then seasoned with fresh or dried herbs and perhaps a little soy sauce. Use three or four different vegetables together, such as broccoli, cauliflower, zucchini, spinach, green beans, snow peas, Chinese cabbage and sprouts. Toss a few sunflower, pumpkin or sesame seeds or a few almonds or pinenuts into the wok with the vegetables and spike with green onions. Make a delicious sauce such as Avocado Dip-Dressing (see page 73) to pour over the top.

You can exchange lunch for dinner, dinner for lunch, if it is more convenient. If you work in an office and take your lunch, prepare a large bag of raw vegetables (carrots, celery, chicory, etc.) and take them with your sprouts to the office along with some seeds and perhaps a jar of avocado sauce or other dressing to dip your vegetables into.

At a restaurant: When you have to eat in a restaurant, ask them to prepare for you an all raw mixed vegetable salad or simply order steamed vegetables without any butter. Then you can have your sprouts in the evening when you are at home.

During the day—throughout the diet—you can drink any variety of herb tea (sweetened, if you like, with honey) as well as fresh fruit and vegetable juices. I find that a drink of vegetable juice can quite easily sustain me when I feel like a snack between meals.

Reorientation—Days 9 and 10 (Saturday and Sunday)

The final two days are designed to adjust your system to a diet containing more cooked food and to set you on the pathway to enjoying a high-raw way of eating afterward. The focus of each meal is still fresh uncooked foods, but one meal a day (lunch or dinner) will contain a cooked dish such as a thick peasant soup, some pulses and/or grains, or a piece of game, poultry or fish.

Days 9 and 10: What to Do
First thing: Wake-up drink as before, and don't forget the skin-brushing!

Breakfast: Birchermuesli with or without yogurt, or a fruit breakfast as on Days 4 to 8.

Lunch: A sprout and vegetable salad as on Days 4 to 8.

Dinner: Crudités or fresh vegetable juice. Then four ounces of poached or grilled fish, or four ounces of chicken roasted without the skin, or a country soup made from beans/grains/lentils and vegetables. Steamed vegetables, brown rice or millet if desired. A green salad. A piece of fresh fruit for dessert (optional).

As with Days 4 to 8, lunch and dinner are interchangeable.

A High-energy, Look-great Way of Living

While you're on the diet social pressures may present stumbling blocks. In Chapter 17 you will find some "aids for survival" which can help you cope with them, as well as a few tips on how to adapt to a permanent high-energy, look-great way of living.

In Chapters 11 to 15 you'll find a few suggestions and guidelines for preparing dishes for the 10-Day Wonder Diet which are delicious, health promoting and beautiful to look at—but make up your own recipes, too, following the principles of the diet. And don't forget to use the ones you like best after your 10-Day Wonder Diet is finished. The Birchermuesli, some of the salads and the Avocado Dip are among my favorite recipes in the world.

I find vegetable bouillon is a great help in many of the dishes of the 10-Day Wonder Diet. The best that I've found is called Morga Vegetable Bouillion, and you can buy it in cube or instant powder form in health food stores and specialty food stores.

11

BREAKFASTS AND DRINKS

Birchermuesli—Swiss Magic

Fruit muesli was originally the invention of the renowned Swiss physician Max Bircher-Benner, who made it famous as part of his effective system of healing based on a high-raw diet. When making muesli you can either use a food processor and do enough for a whole family at once or, with a simple hand grater, make one bowlful. But be sure to experiment with all the many variations depending on what kind of fruits are in season. Each has its own delicious character.

Birchermuesli (for one)

2 tbsp oatflakes (or a combination of oat, rye, wheat, etc.) soaked overnight in a little water or fruit juice (e.g., pineapple)
1 apple or firm pear, grated
a handful of soaked raisins
1/2 lemon
2 tbsp plain yogurt
1 tbsp minced nuts (e.g., almonds and brazils)
1 tsp honey, cinnamon or powdered ginger

Soak the flakes with the raisins overnight in a little water or fruit juice. Combine with this mixture a grated apple or pear with a squeeze of lemon juice and one or two tablespoonfuls of natural plain yogurt. Drizzle with honey if desired (the dish is beautifully sweet even without it) and sprinkle with chopped nuts and cinnamon or ginger.

The above recipe calls for an apple or pear, but you can use almost any other fruit instead, or add extra fruit in season:

Banana Muesli: Add a banana sliced in quarters lengthwise and then chopped crosswise into small pieces. Or mash a banana with a little yogurt or fruit juice and use as a topping.

Summer Muesli: Add a handful of raspberries, strawberries, black currants or pitted cherries to the basic muesli, or substitute a finely diced peach or nectarine in place of the apple or pear.

Winter Muesli: Soak overnight in water a selection of dried fruits such as apricots, raisins, figs, dates and pears. Dice into small pieces or cut up with a pair of scissors, and add to the other muesli ingredients. Spice with a pinch of nutmeg.

Dairy-free Muesli: In place of the yogurt use some fresh fruit juice such as apple, orange or grape. To thicken the juice, blend with a little fresh fruit such as banana, pear or apple.

Shakes

Fruit Shake

> *1 cup plain yogurt*
> *1 ripe banana*
> *few drops vanilla extract*
> *1 tsp honey*
> *1 tsp coconut (optional)*

Combine the ingredients thoroughly in a blender. As a variation, try replacing the banana with a handful of berries, half a papaya or mango, or a few chunks of fresh pineapple.

Nut-milk Shakes

These are the dairy-free alternatives to the fruit shake. For the basic recipe use:

1/3 cup almonds (blanched)
2/3 cup water
5 pitted dates
few drops vanilla extract
1 tsp honey

Blend the water and the almonds really well until the mixture is smooth. If you have used unblanched almonds, strain the mixture at this stage to remove the ground up husks. Add the other ingredients and process well. Serve immediately.

Apricot Shake: Use apricots, fresh or dried, instead of the dates, and add a handful of sunflower seeds to the nuts before you blend.

Grape Shake: Use fruit juice such as grape or apple instead of the water, and raisins instead of the dates. Omit the honey and vanilla if desired.

For extra goodness add a teaspoonful of brewers' yeast (the de-bittered kind is the most bearable), a tablespoonful of wheatgerm, or the yolk of an egg. Blend well.

Instant Low-fat Yogurt

If you are using yogurt, why not try making your own? It's very simple and doesn't require a lot of expensive equipment. The easiest way to make it is in a wide-mouthed flask, but an earthenware crock or dish kept in a warm place will do just as well.

One of the very simplest methods of making yogurt is to use low-fat skimmed milk powder. Mix up two pints of milk using one and a half times the amount of powdered milk suggested on the packet. If you use boiling water from a

kettle and add cold water to it you can get just the temperature of milk you need and don't have to bother heating your
milk in a saucepan. Add two tablespoonfuls of plain yogurt
as a "starter" and leave in a suitable container which will
retain the heat (such as a Thermos bottle) for about eight
hours.

Herb Teas

A simple herb tea is light and refreshing and can either be
drunk hot with a little honey for sweetening or made double-
strength, chilled and served with mint and a slice of lemon in
a tall iced glass.

Herb teas make seductive but healthy alternatives to tea
and coffee. They come in two varieties: those which you
drink for medicinal purposes—such as sage for a sore throat,
dandelion to eliminate excess water from the body, lemon
grass for indigestion, and St. John's Wort for skin problems—and those which you drink for pure pleasure. Some
herb teas, such as camomile and vervain which are natural
sedatives and peppermint which calms the digestive system,
belong in both categories. Some of my favorites include
lemon grass, lemon verbena, orange blossom, hibiscus and
linden blossom.

You can make your own from dried herbs, or you can
buy herb teas ready packaged in bags which you use as you
would ordinary tea bags—allowing them a little longer to
steep. There are some wonderful herbal combinations on the
market in these little bags—cinnamon-and-rose flavor, for
instance, or apple-and-cinnamon. Or you can drink single-
herb teas.

To Make Herb Teas
Take about a tablespoonful of the dried herbs (either a single
herb or a mixture) to make two cups. Pour boiling water over
the herbs and let them steep in a pot for 5–10 minutes,
stirring every now and then to extract the full aroma. Now

strain and serve with a slice of lemon and/or a little honey for sweetening.

Other Drinks

Aside from the herb teas, the only other drinks you should think of taking while on the 10-Day Wonder Diet are water and fruit and vegetable juices.

The water which you drink should be either filtered or spring water, and certainly *not* just tap water, which contains all sorts of chemical additives your body can well do without.

Similarly, don't just drink any fruit or vegetable juice: a lot of the ones you find in the shops have additives, are reconstituted from concentrated or frozen juices—or aren't really juices at all but flavored drinks! You can make your own with a juice extractor, or you can look out for commercial ones where the processing has been done at low temperatures. Juices marketed under the label Biotta are good.

12

SPROUTS AND SALADS

$\mathbb{T}$here are so many delicious ways of using raw vegetables that it would be hard to list them all. Let's start by looking at how to sprout and then at some salad suggestions.

Sprouting

When a seed is sprouted its vitamin content increases by up to 700 percent—sprouts even contain vitamin B_{12} (very few vegetables have this one). During the sprouting process starch begins to be broken down into simple sugars, fats to fatty acids, and proteins to amino acids (the ratio of essential amino acids to non-essential ones even increases). Because of this the seed is already, as it were, partially digested and therefore very easily assimilated. Remarkably, a grain even loses its mucus-inducing properties when sprouted.

Sprouts are the finest rejuvenating foods available. They are simple to grow, taste delicious and, what's more, they're cheap. All you need to start your own indoor germinating "factory" are a few old jars, some pure water, fresh seeds/beans/grains and a warm spot in the kitchen.

Sprouters
A home-made sprouter can be anything from a bucket to a polythene bag, but the best ones are wide-mouthed glass jars. Some people like to make a neat sprouter by covering the jar with cheesecloth, nylon or wire mesh and securing it

with a rubber band, or using a mason jar with a screw-on rim to hold the cheesecloth in place. The easiest and least fussy way is simply to use open jars and cover a row of them with a tea towel to prevent dust and insects getting in.

Good sprouts to start with are those from mung beans, brown lentils, fenugreek seeds, alfalfa seeds and chickpeas.

To Begin

1. Put the seeds/beans/grains of your choice (for example, mung) in a large sieve. (For the amount to use see the chart—remember most sprouts give a volume about eight times that of the dry beans.) Remove any small stones, broken seeds or loose husks and rinse the sprouts well.
2. Put the seeds/beans/grains in a jar and cover with a few inches of pure water. (Rinsing can be done in tap water, but the initial soak, when the seeds absorb a lot of water to set their enzymes in action, is best done in spring, filtered or boiled water, as the chlorine in tap water can sometimes inhibit germination.)
3. Leave the sprouts in a warm place to soak overnight or as long as is needed (see chart).
4. Pour off the soak-water. If none remains then you still have thirsty seeds/beans/grains on your hands, so give them more water to absorb.
5. Rinse the seeds/beans/grains, either by pouring water through the cheesecloth top, swishing it around and pouring it off several times, or by tipping them from the open-topped jars into a large sieve and rinsing them well under the tap before replacing them. Whichever way you do it, be sure that they are well drained, as too much water may cause them to rot. The cheesecloth covered jars can be left tilted in a dish drainer to allow all the water to run out. Repeat this every morning and night.
6. After about 3–5 days the sprouts are ready to eat. Rinse them and pop them into polythene bags and then store them in the refrigerator for use in your salads. Most sprouts will keep fresh in a refrigerator for from 5 to 7 days this way.

SPROUTING CHART

Small Seeds soak 6–8 hrs. except as stated	Dry amount to yield 1 liter (1¾ pints)	Ready to eat in	Length of shoot (approx.)	Growing tips and notes
Alfalfa	3–4T	5–6 days	3.5 cm (1½ in)	Rich in organic vitamins and minerals, the roots of the mature plant penetrate the earth to a depth of 10–30 m (30–100 ft).
Fenugreek	½C	3–4 days	1 cm (½ in)	Has quite a strong "curry" taste. Best mixed with other sprouts. Good for ridding the body of toxins.
Mustard no soaking needed	¼C	4–5 days	2.5 cm (1 in)	Can be grown on damp paper towels for a week or more. The green tops are then cut off with scissors and used in salads.
Radish no soaking needed	¼C	4–5 days	2.5 cm (1 in)	The red-hot flavor is great for dressings, or mixed with other sprouts. Good for clearing mucus and healing mucous membranes.
Sesame	½C	1–2 days	Same length as seed	If grown for longer than about two days sesame sprouts become very bitter.
LARGER SEEDS soak 10–15 hrs.	To yield 2 liters (3½ pints)			
Aduki (adzuki) beans	1½C	3–5 days	2.5–3.5 cm (1–1½ in)	Have a nutty "legume" flavor. Especially good for the kidneys.
Chick peas	2C	3–4 days	2.5 cm (1 in)	May need to soak for about 18 hours to swell to their full size. The water should be renewed twice during this time.

Lentils	1C	3–5 days	0.5–2.5 cm (1/4–1 in)	Try all different kinds of lentils—red, Chinese, green, brown. They are good eaten young or up to about 6 days old.
Mung beans	1C	3–5 days	1–5 cm (1/2–2 1/2 in)	Soak at least 15 hours. Keep in the dark for a sweet sprout.
Soya beans	1C	3–5 days	3.5 cm (1 1/2 in)	Need to soak for up to 24 hours with frequent changes of water to prevent fermentation. Remove any damaged beans which fail to germinate.
Sunflower	4C	1–2 days	Same length as seed	Can be grown for their greens. When using sunflower seeds soak them and sprout for just a day. They bruise easily so handle with care.

GRAINS

soak 12–15 hrs. except as stated

To yield 1 liter (1 3/4 pints)

Wheat	2C	2–3 days	Same length as grain	An excellent source of the B vitamins. The soak water can be drunk straight, added to soups and vegetable juices or fermented to make rejuvelac.
Rye	2C	2–3 days	Same length as grain	Has a delicious distinctive flavor. Good for the glandular system.
Barley	2C	2–3 days	Same length as grain	As with most sprouts, barley becomes quite sweet when germinated. Particularly good for people who are weak or underweight.
Oats soak 5–8 hrs only	2C	3–4 days	Same length as grain	You need whole oats or "oat groats." Oats lose much of their mucus-forming activity when sprouted.
Millet soak 5–8 hrs only	2C	3–4 days	Same length as grain	Must be unhulled millet. The only grain that is alkaline.

Salads
Here are some salad suggestions—salads which you can make in one dish for one person and which are meals in themselves. But do experiment using different combinations of root, leaf and bulb vegetables—whatever are available in the shops—to make up your own recipes as well.

The appearance of any salad is important. Fortunately the brilliant colors of fresh vegetables and fruits are quite stunning. It is nice to experiment with different decorative ways of chopping fruits and vegetables to make attractive garnishes.

Red Devil Salad
Make a base of radicchio (or any other lettuce) leaves to line the dish. On this arrange in segments:

> grated carrot placed inside a ring of red pepper and topped with a few fresh garden peas
> a small bunch of watercress inside a ring of sweet yellow pepper
> half an avocado (brush with lemon juice or olive oil to prevent its going brown) filled with radish slices
> a handful of Chinese (mung) bean sprouts
> a few diagonal slices of cucumber
> a few cauliflower and broccoli florets
> some grated raw beetroot
> some grated white radish
> mustard greens and cress
> a tomato sliced into segments but not all the way through, so that it looks like a flower with its petals open

Festival Salad
Line the bowl with Chinese cabbage leaves and in it put:

> celery and carrot sticks looped through rings of bell peppers
> a few slices of fennel
> a few slices of baby turnip (raw)
> some snow peas
> some slices of apple
> slices of red onion

SPROUTS AND SALADS ■ *69*

radish roses (made by cutting zigzags around the middle of the
  radish and separating the two halves)
a small bunch of grapes
watercress and parsley
an orange sliced in segments with the skin left on for decoration,
  but peeled back in sections so that it can easily be removed
a handful of chickpea sprouts

Sprout Magic Salad
Make a base with alfalfa sprouts, and around the dish arrange:

  grated carrot
  red cabbage
  white cabbage
  beetroot

  Add:

  sliced mushrooms
  black olives
  green onions

Sprinkle raisins over the grated vegetables and add a spoon-
ful of seed or nut cheese.

Spinach with a Difference
Make a base by shredding tender spinach leaves finely (remove the stalks), and on it arrange:

  a handful of baby button mushrooms with their stems trimmed
  half an avocado diced (simply slice the flesh in its shell several
    times first vertically and then horizontally, and then scoop
    out the flesh with a spoon)
  some diced red pepper
  apple rings (remove the core from the apple and slice crosswise)
  thin slices of Jerusalem artichoke, kohlrabi or new potatoes
    (raw)
  toasted pumpkin seeds

Red and Yellow Wonder

shredded iceberg lettuce base
thin slices of carrot and zucchini (the slicer attachment on a food
    processor is ideal for this)
a few cherry tomatoes
sweetcorn—scraped raw off the cob, or cooked on the cob
a few toasted hazelnuts
mustard greens and cress

13

DRESSINGS

You can make a simple dressing by mixing herbs and mustard with a little yogurt (the thicker the yogurt the better) or you can explore some of the beauty of classic oil-based dressings instead. Oil dressings are especially good for leafy salads such as those in which lettuce and spinach predominate. With the right seasonings, such as a tasty mustard and/or various herbs, they can be very flavorful and not at all the plain "oil-and-vinegar-dressing" most people know.

Basic French Dressing

3/4 cup oil
1/4 cup lemon juice or cider vinegar
1 tsp whole-grain mustard (French Meaux mustard is my favorite) or mustard powder
2 tsp honey
a little vegetable bouillon powder and pepper to season
a small clove of crushed garlic (optional)

Combine all the ingredients in a blender or simply place in a screw-top jar and shake well to mix. Some people like to thin the dressing and make it a little lighter by adding a couple of tablespoonfuls of water.

Here are some suggestions for dressings beginning with the French dressing base.

Rich French dressing: To the basic recipe add:

> *1 tbsp tamari sauce*
> *1 finely chopped scallion*
> *dash of cayenne pepper*

Wine dressing: To the basic recipe add 1 tablespoonful of red or white wine—white is good for salads containing fruit, red for cabbage salads.

Herb dressing: My favorite combination of herbs for dressing is:

> *marjoram*
> *basil*
> *thyme*
> *dill*
> *mint*

You need about 3–4 tablespoonfuls in all of fresh, finely chopped herbs, or 2 teaspoonfuls of dried.

Citrus dressing: In the basic dressing recipe use:

> *3/4 cup sesame oil*
> *juice of 1/2 lemon and 1 orange*
> *1 tbsp vinegar*

> *Add:*

> *1 tsp grated orange peel and 1/2 tsp grated lemon peel (scrub the fruits first!)*
> *pinch of nutmeg*
> *1 tsp chervil*

Put all the ingredients in the blender and combine until smooth.

Spicy Italian dressing: Follow the basic recipe using cider vinegar and add:

> *dash of red wine or tamari sauce*
> *2 ripe peeled tomatoes*

1 tbsp finely chopped onion or garlic
¹/₂ tsp oregano and basil
powdered bay leaf

Blend all the ingredients well.

Olive dressing: Use olive oil and lemon juice in the basic recipe, and add:

4–6 pitted black olives (finely chopped)
pinch of cayenne pepper

Avocado Dip or Dressing
This is my favorite of all salad dressings. You can make it thick as a dip for crudités or thin to pour over a salad.

1–2 avocados
1 cup fresh orange juice (use more or less to give the desired consistency)
1 tsp curry powder
2 tsp vegetable bouillon powder
fresh herbs (parsley, dill)
1 small clove garlic (optional)

Peel and pit the avocado(s). Blend all the ingredients together in a food processor until smooth.

14

GRAINS AND PULSES

Grains and pulses are wonderful natural staples. Let's look at the grains first.

Brown rice, wheat, barley, oats, millet, bulgar wheat and buckwheat are superb staple foods—high in fiber, a good source of protein when eaten with vegetables, and very filling. They are exceptionally useful for athletes and for people who want to have sustained energy.

How do you serve grains? There are so many delicious ways. On their own with a few herbs tossed in, with a few vegetables such as onions and mushrooms, and in thick nourishing country soups. Cold leftover grains can be mixed into salads.

The basic rule for cooking grains is that you need about half a cup of dry whole grains to serve each person.

Wash the grains in cool water, using a strainer to gently loosen the dust and small bits of dirt. Check to see there are no little bits of rock left. When the water rinses through the strainer clean, the grains are ready to cook.

There are two basic ways of cooking whole or cracked grains. The first uses cold water mixed with the grain; in the second you add boiling water to the grain.

I usually prefer the boiling-water method. Sauté the grain either in a heavy dry pan or with the smallest possible amount of olive oil to brown it a little; this is not necessary with rice or barley, but the others benefit greatly from it. Now add boiling water (for guides to quantity see below), a handful of herbs and some vegetable bouillon powder to the pot and cover immediately. Bring to the boil and continue to cook at simmer on the burner or (I prefer this) pop it all into a moderate oven to finish (see notes on times below). Do not stir the grains as this breaks them up and makes them stick in clumps.

Every grain needs a slightly different length of cooking time; the amount of water needed varies too. Here are some guidelines.

Brown rice: Use twice as much water as rice and cook for 45 minutes. Usually I cook rice by simply adding cold water to the grain, bringing to the boil, and then simmering.

Millet and buckwheat groats: Use one part grain to two parts water and cook for 20–25 minutes. Millet can be cooked using the cold-water method.

Bulgar wheat: This is wheat which has been cracked, toasted and steamed before you buy it. Use one part bulgar wheat to one and a half parts water. Cook for 20 minutes.

Barley: Use twice as much water as grain and cook for 90 minutes.

The Humble Pulses

One cup of beans, lentils or peas measured dry makes about four average servings. Like the grains, these inexpensive foods are rich in fiber and have good sustaining power. And they come in such wonderful varieties—black beans, lima beans, kidney beans, soy beans, lentils of all sorts and colors, aduki (adzuki) beans and chickpeas. I use them as the base for delicious soups and casserole dishes with them lavished with fresh herbs; I also mix them with salads sometimes.

Here's how to cook the pulses. Unless they are very dirty, they need only one rinse under running water before cooking. I usually soak pulses for several hours—or overnight—in a cool place before cooking them. This softens them and cuts the cooking time considerably. It also helps break down some of the starches they contain and renders them more digestible. After soaking, put them in a pot, add three times as much water as pulses, bring to the boil and simmer until done; remember that kidney beans *must* be boiled for at least 10 minutes, as otherwise they're poisonous. Like grains, pulses can be cooked in the oven instead of on top of the burner. I prefer oven cooking because you don't have to be so accurate about the time you take them out and because they are less likely to stick to the pot. Beans and lentils love carrots, onions and celery, which I often add—as well as herbs and seasoning. (Vegetable bouillon powder works its magic here as well.)

Here's a brief guide to timings:

RED LENTILS	20 minutes *(don't need soaking either)*
SPLIT PEAS AND OTHER LENTILS:	one hour
OTHERS (except soy beans):	one and a half hours
SOY BEANS:	two and a half hours
CHICKPEAS:	one and a half hours

15

SOUPS AND WOKS

The winter soups in this chapter are hearty and full-bodied. I make them from whatever vegetables I happen to have, adding some millet, lentils, peas, rice, barley or whatever is handy for thickening, lots of fresh herbs from the garden or a few dried herbs, and perhaps some bouillon powder for seasoning.

Thick Vegetable Soup

1 large onion
2 leeks
1 head of celery
4 carrots
2 turnips
1 parsnip
any other vegetable you happen to have or want to substitute
2 tbsp olive oil
3 pints stock or water (boiling)
1 tbsp bouillon powder
2 bay leaves
3/4 cup brown rice or millet
2 cups green peas
1 cup string beans
fresh parsley

Wash and peel the vegetables and peel the onions. Cut root vegetables into small cubes—the leeks first lengthwise 4 to 6 times and then across so that you get tiny pieces. Add oil to the pot and sauté the leeks. Then add chopped celery, carrots, turnips and parsnip; put the lid on and allow them to sweat for five minutes. Now add your boiling stock or water, the vegetable bouillon, the bay leaves and the rice or millet and allow to cook for 30 minutes. Now add peas and beans and cook for another 15 minutes. Sprinkle with chopped parsley and serve.

This makes enough for a large family—4 to 6 good-size servings.

Borscht

   3 raw beetroots (with their green tops, if possible)
   3 carrots
   1 medium onion
   1/2 small cabbage
   2 tbsp olive oil
   2 pints stock or water (boiling)
   1 tbsp vegetable bouillon powder
   juice of one lemon
   3 tbsp honey
   dash of nutmeg
   1 cup thick yogurt or sour cream

Wash vegetables—do not peel—and cut them into small strips. Retain half of one beetroot which you will add grated to the soup later. Heat oil in pot and sweat beetroot and onions for five minutes, then add the rest of the vegetables, including the sliced beet greens (if you have them), and stew for another 5–10 minutes stirring occasionally. Add stock or water—boiling—together with bouillon powder, and cook vegetables until tender. Now add lemon juice, grated beetroot and honey and cook for another 5 minutes. Serve topped with the thick yogurt or sour cream and sprinkle with nutmeg.

Serves 4 to 6 people well.

Potato Soup

6 medium potatoes
2¹/₂ pints water or stock
1 tbsp vegetable bouillon powder
1 cup sliced, chunked or diced vegetables (e.g., leeks, celery, carrot, swede, green beans, peas)
herbs (e.g., marjoram, winter savory, basil, garlic)
garnishes (e.g., sliced green onions, chopped hard-boiled egg, chives, watercress, grated hard cheese)

Wash vegetables and scrub potatoes, cutting them into medium-sized chunks. Cover the potatoes in the water or stock to which the bouillon has been added and boil until tender. Remove from heat and blend in a food processor until smooth. Now sauté the vegetables and cut into small pieces, add them along with your seasonings to the potato mixture, and cook for five minutes. Sprinkle with your garnishes and serve.

Serves 4 to 6 people.

Wok Frying

The most delicious way of all to cook vegetables is *à la Chinoise*—in a wok or simple frying pan. It is quick, simple and a lot of fun to do. Here's how.

Take whatever vegetables you happen to have. A good combination would be:

2 tbsp vegetable oil
handful of cashew nuts
onions cut in rings
cauliflower broken into florets
spiked green onions (their green parts slit lengthwise)
snow peas
diced red pepper
sliced mushrooms
tamari or soy sauce

Put the oil into your pan and heat. Add cashews on their own and brown, then add vegetables which take longest to cook such as onions and cauliflower. Sauté for two to three minutes turning constantly. Now add the rest of the vegetables and continue to toss them in the pan for another three to five minutes. Add a little tamari soy sauce and serve.

16

STEP BY STEP

Making the 10-Day Plan work for you is simply a matter of putting the tools for detoxification outlined in this little book into a daily program which you can fit into your own lifestyle and the demands made upon your time. And you needn't go on vacation to some blissful peaceful spot for it all to happen, either. With a little forethought you will be able to manage it pleasantly and easily at home without interfering with your work, family duties or anything else. Of course, there are a few changes which you may need to make to accommodate the special demands you'll be making on your body during this special 10-day period. For instance, you will need to postpone that dinner party or going out for drinks—that is, unless you can order a mineral water. Also you will want to see that you can get to bed most nights reasonably early. For the process of spring-cleaning the body is a dynamic one which can use up a lot of energy in itself. During this 10-day period it is a good idea to get as much rest as possible so your body can begin to renew itself.

Just how you arrange your schedule depends upon your circumstances, but it is a good idea to sit down for a few minutes the day before you begin the 10-Day Plan and make yourself a personal daily schedule which will enable you to fit everything in comfortably. Hang it in your closet or on the inside of a kitchen cupboard so you can refer to it whenever you need to for guidance. Just to give you some idea, here is what mine tends to look like (but remember I am an early riser and have long been a slow but addicted runner). Yours will probably be quite different. You will see that my schedule has lots of little gaps of five or ten minutes in it. These are the times in which I do things like read the newspaper, get changed, or simply . . . putter around!

5:30	Wake up. Do five to ten minutes of gentle deep breathing while still in bed.
5:45	Get up
5:50–6:05	Skin-brushing and a shower
6:15–8:00	Work
8:00–8:30	Breakfast
9:00–12:15	Work
12:30–12:45	Relaxation response
1:00–1:30	Lunch
1:45–5:15	Work
5:30–6:30	Running for 40 minutes, then a shower
7:00	Supper, then evening free (evenings 1, 6 and 10 of the 10-Day Plan I take a sauna at the local health club)
10:00	Sleep

Once you have worked out your own plan then try to stick to it. It can be a lot of fun to carry out the 10-Day Plan with your mate or a friend; then you have company and can help each other. Chances are, when those around you see just how much these simple natural techniques for spring-cleaning have done for you, they will want to join in too.

I use the 10-Day Plan at least twice a year—once in the spring, which is the traditional time for detoxifying the body, and whenever I feel particularly jaded or tired from having worked too hard, eaten too much or been forced to live on hotel food for a couple of weeks at a time. I have been doing it for more than 15 years and yet each time I am constantly amazed at just how wonderful it can make me feel.

But the 10-Day Plan is only the beginning of a whole new you. What comes after matters most of all.

17

NEW LIFE STARTS HERE

Do you wake up most mornings feeling great? Or is it a monumental effort just to lift your head off the pillow? Having energy to spare for fun after a long day's work at home or away can be a lot easier to achieve than you might imagine. You can arrive at work bright and energetic every morning and go home with vitality to spare. Or you can cope with young children, a house, shopping and all the rest and still be fit for enjoyment in the evenings provided you build yourself a lifestyle for high-level fitness and health.

The 10-Day Plan is a wonderful way to set you on the road. But it is only the beginning. After completing it you need to start thinking about how to develop a high-energy lifestyle. It can be a lot easier than you might imagine. It probably only means making a few changes in the way you do things now and incorporating a couple of the 10-Day techniques—such as exercising and destressing—into your daily life. For instance, get yourself out to walk for 30 to 45 minutes every morning, rain or shine—if necessary before everybody else is up.

And steal 10 to 15 minutes twice a day to practice the relaxation technique you have learned. You can do it on a bus or train to work, or simply lock yourself in a room when the children have gone to bed. What's important is that you do it regularly every day. For it is this imprinting of the technique on your consciousness from daily repetition which makes it such a powerful tool for health and emotional balance. You may think that you just don't have time because of all the demands on your life. The truth is that none of us *has* time. Each of us has to *make* time. And, whatever your personal circumstances, you are not alone in having demands made upon you. We all have them. Like many people, I have raised four children on my own and had to run a house and work full-time. If it hadn't been for the strength I've gained from stealing time for regular exercise and destressing, I would never have been able to do it. For the time you take repays itself tenfold in the energy you gain from it and in the way in which both exercise and relaxation make it possible for you to do more work, more efficiently and with less wasted effort. But exercise and destressing are not enough on their own. Probably the most important thing of all for vitality and health is how you eat.

Eat to Live

What you eat (or *don't* eat) for breakfast can have a lot to do with whether, after a long day, you are still full of bounce or ready to collapse in a heap. Many people think that when they are tired—say, first thing in the morning or around 11 o'clock, or in mid-afternoon—what they need is a sweet roll, a chocolate bar or a cup of coffee to pep them up. It is true that, because of the way these things act on your body's chemistry, they can bring a quick boost. The only catch is that the boost comes at a price to your overall health, vitality and good looks. For, while sweet food or a cup of coffee will temporarily pep you up, it can let you down with a crash a couple of hours later. And, if you eat sweets or drink coffee regularly, as many people do, they can seriously interfere with your energy levels by disrupting the delicate mechanisms which regulate your blood sugar. They can also make you dependent on them just to keep going—a dependency no really fit person wants or needs.

Go for the Steady Sustainers

The best foods to eat for real energy and lasting health are not the "quick boosters" full of sugar and caffeine but the "steady sustainers"—fresh natural foods as our grandparents knew them: fresh fruits and vegetables, wholegrain cereals and wholemeal bread—high in natural fiber—spread with a little of the best butter. Simply prepared and eaten wherever possible in their whole state (remember to eat the skin of your baked potato and the peel of your apple), these foods, plus a small quantity of good-quality animal protein such as fish or chicken or game if you like (the latest research shows you are best off without *too* much), offer the best guarantee of high-level health and vitality you will find anywhere.

Don't much care for breakfast? OK: Don't skip it, though, or you will experience an "energy slump" later in the day. It needn't take long or be complicated. Make yourself something natural and simple. Eat a piece of fresh fruit and a slice of 100 percent whole-wheat toast spread with butter and perhaps a little honey. Or make yourself a quick bowl of muesli or one of the sustaining breakfast drinks you've learned about in Chapter 11.

Such a breakfast will lift your energy levels without ever letting you down thanks to the natural goodness of the fruit or the drink. Also, the complex carbohydrates plus the high fiber content of whole-grain bread release a steady stream of energy into your bloodstream to keep you gliding through the morning without fatigue. If you find yourself hungry between meals or if you are feeling a bit tired during the day, try munching a handful of natural, unsalted sunflower seeds or an apple or a small bunch of grapes instead of a pastry or sweets.

To stay well and full of energy long after you've finished your 10-Day Plan, make one meal a day a large salad complete with all the delicious trimmings and trappings you have come to know from the diet. And choose all of your other foods from the natural, wholesome "energy-maker" foods rather than the refined and over-processed "energy-breaker" foods. Taken along with all the health-giving benefits of your new exercise program, eating like this will mean that you'll very quickly find yourself feeling terrific. Here are a few guidelines.

The Energy Makers

fresh vegetables—especially eaten raw
fresh fruits
100 percent whole-grain bread—dark and delicious
wholegrain cereals such as muesli and granola (but read the labels and watch out for hidden sugars in these)
fresh fruit juices
pulses
low-fat cheeses like cottage cheese, ricotta and Edam
eggs
fish
chicken
game

The Energy Breakers

white bread, rolls, pastries and pies
pasta—spaghetti, macaroni, etc.
sugar and anything containing it
biscuits made from white flour
jelly
jams
canned fruits
packet and canned soups
french fries
potato chips
fizzy drinks containing sugar or artificial sweeteners
greasy fried foods
chocolate and sweets
artificial fruit drinks

A Fitter, More Healthy Lifestyle Starts Here

These three little tricks—a daily exercise program of simply walking briskly for 30 to 45 minutes or doing some other form of rhythmic exercise, a diet rich in natural unprocessed foods, and the daily practice of a simple relaxation technique such as the relaxation response (see Chapter 9)—can be nothing less than revolutionary to how you look and feel.

Reading about them is only the first step. What really matters is getting started. The 10-Day Plan comes first. But that is only the beginning, to set you on the road to a new lifestyle for vitality, good looks and long-lasting health. In time, all of these tools for health and energy can become so much a part of your life that they become habits. Then you may never have to give a thought to your health again.

That, after all, is what being really healthy is all about.

INDEX

Page numbers in **boldface** refer to major discussions

89